This Colouring Book Belongs to:

_____

_____

Right tibia and fibula posterior View (Right Side)

1. Fibular articular
2. Medial malleolus
3. Groove for tibialis posterior tendon
4. Shaft of tibia
5. Posterior surface
6. Medial Border
7. Nutrient foramen
8. Soleal line
9. Posterior intercondylar area
10. Medial condyle
11. Medial tibial plateau
12. Intercondylar tubercles of intercondylar eminence
13. Lateral tibial plateau
14. Lateral condyle
15. Apex of head
16. Head of fibula (contacting fibular articular facet of tibia)
17. Medial crest
18. interosseous membrane
19. interosseous border
20. Posterior border
21. Fibular notch of tibia, occupied by fibula
22. Lateral malleolus

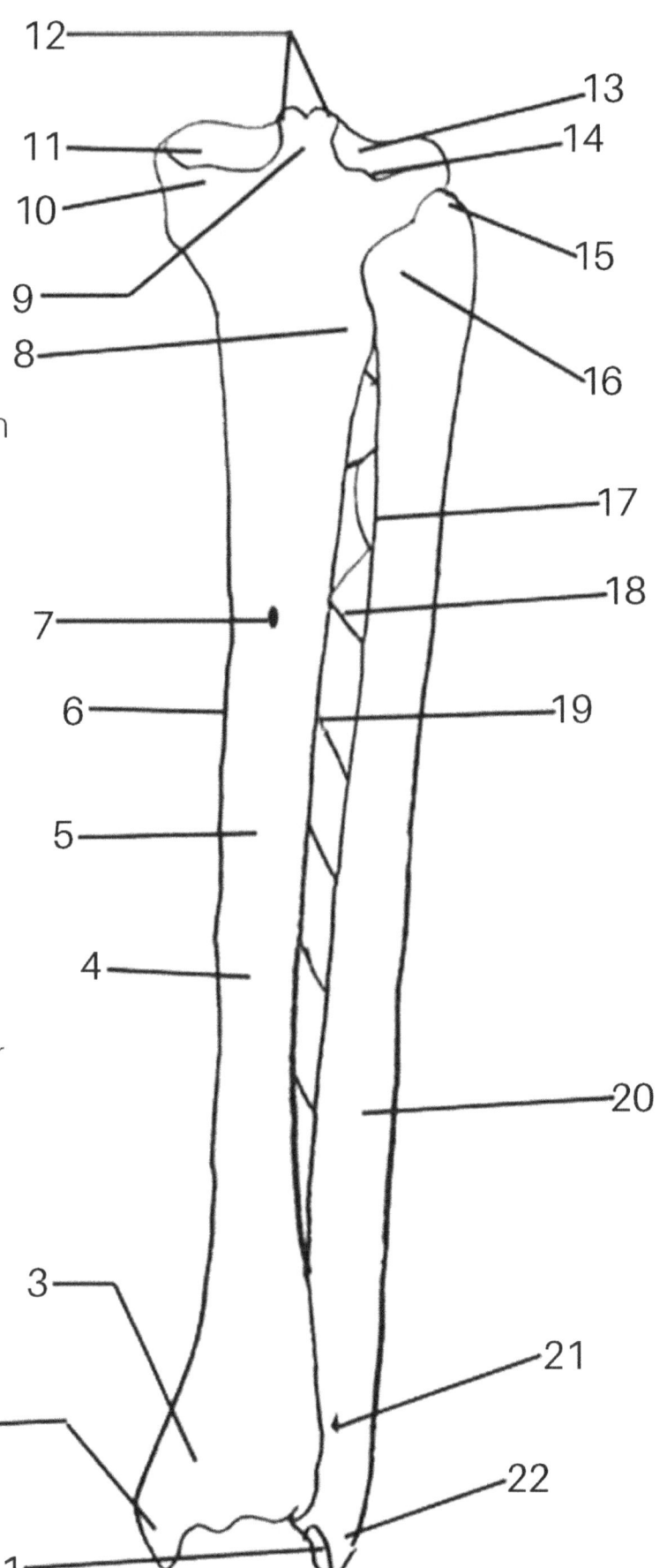

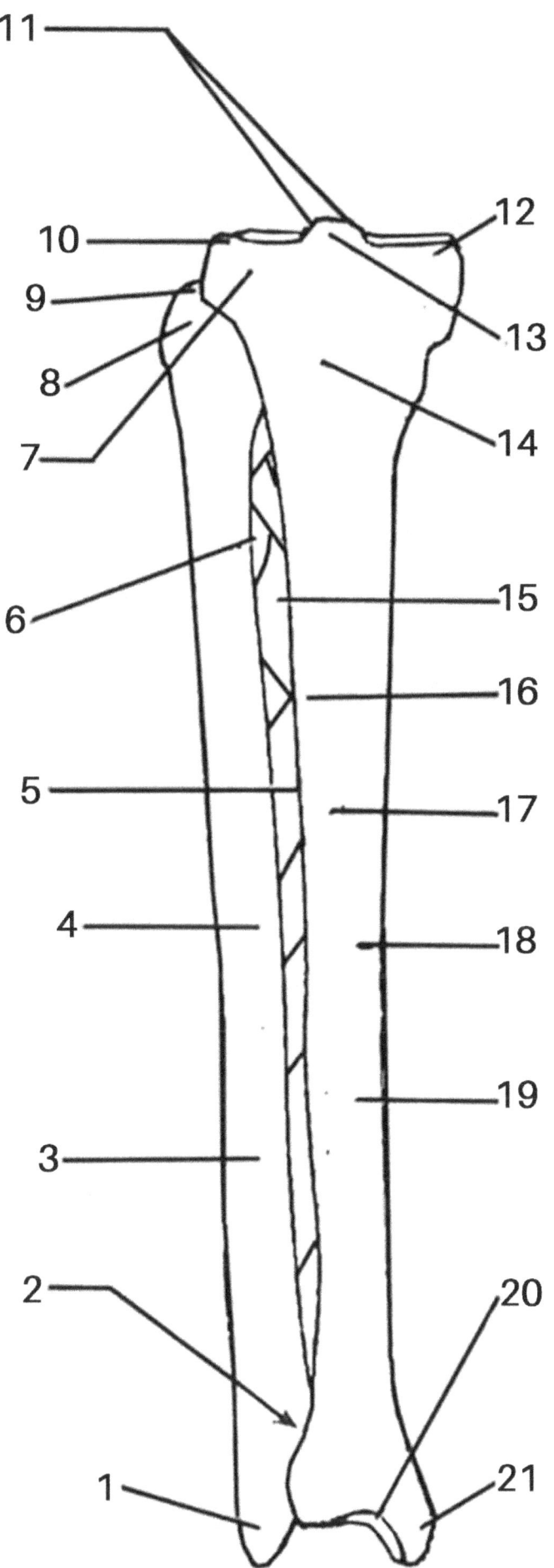

Right Tibia and Fibula (Anterior View)

1. Lateral malleolus
2. Fibular notch of tibia occupied by fibula
3. Shaft of fibula
4. Anterior border
5. Interosseous border
6. Opening for arterior tibial vessels
7. Anterolateral tibial (Gerdy) tubercle
8. Head of fibula
9. Apex of head
10. Lateral condyle
11. Intercondylar tubercles of intercondylar eminence
12. Medial condyle
13. Anterior intercondylar area
14. Tibial tuberosity
15. Interosseous membrane
16. Lateral surface
17. Anterior border
18. Medial surface
19. Shaft (body) of tibia
20. Tibial articular surface
21. Medial malleolus

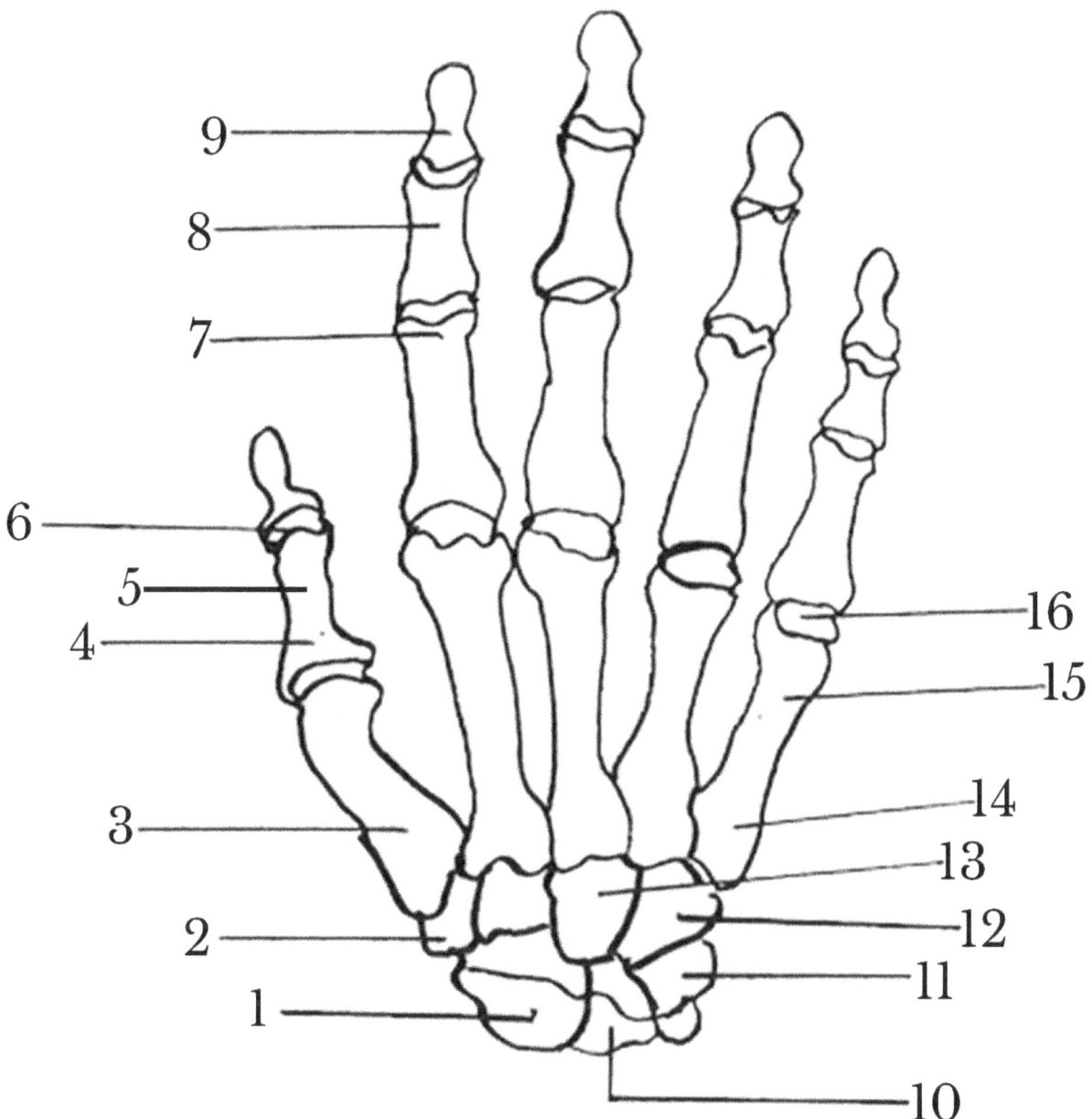

Bone of Right Hand
Anterior (Palmar) View

1. Scaphoid
2. Trapezium (Tz)
3. 1st metacarpal
4. Base
5. Shaft
6. Head
7. Proximal ⎫
8. Middle   ⎬ Phalanges
9. Distal   ⎭
10. Lunate
11. Triquetrum
12. Hamate (H)
13. Capitate
14. Base
15. Shaft
16. Head

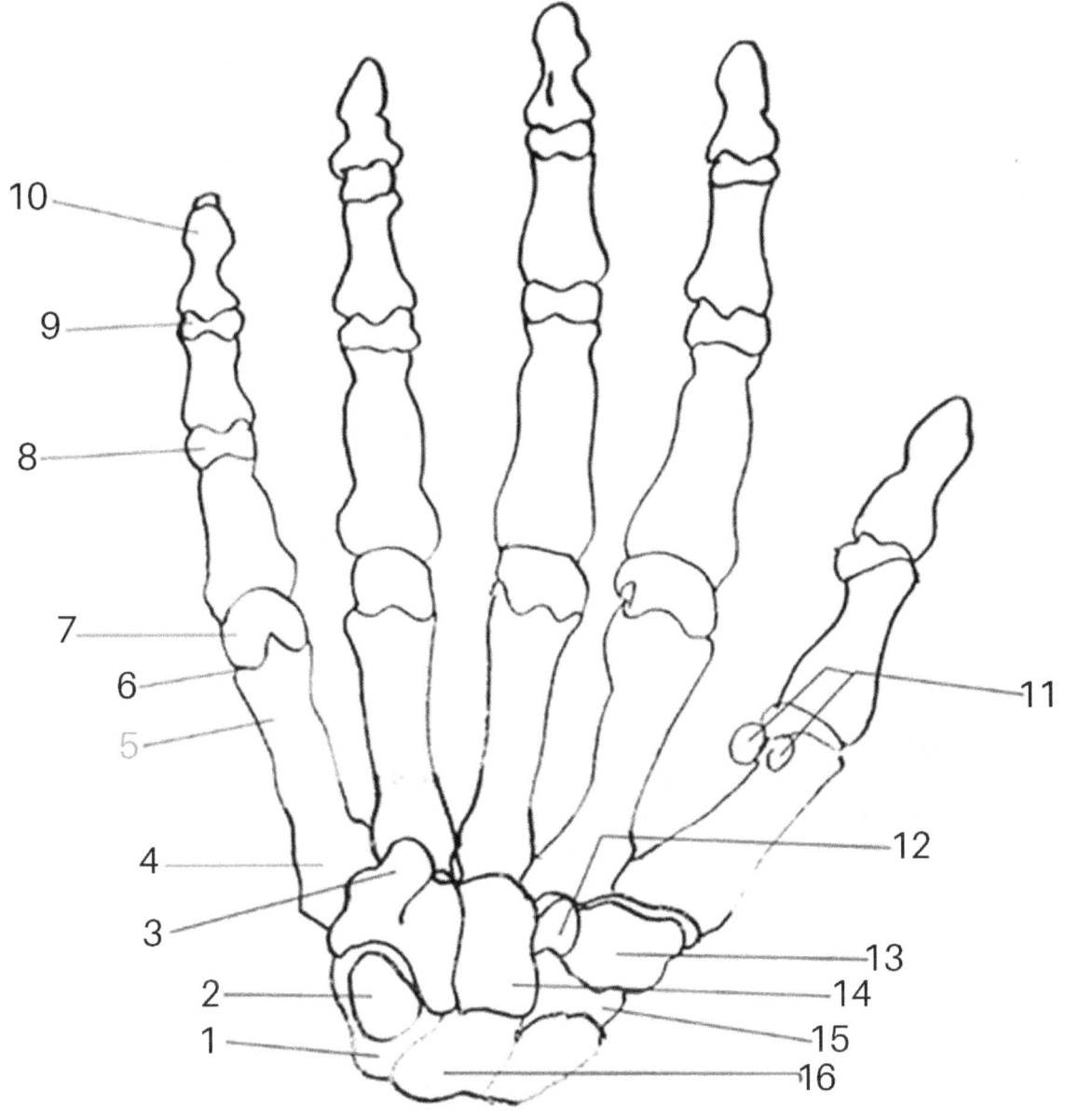

Bones of Right Hand - Anterior (Palmer) View

1. Triquetrum (Tq)
2. Pisiform (P)
3. Hook of hamate
4. Base
5. Shaft
6. Tubercle } 5th metacarpal
7. Head
8. Head of proximal phalanx
9. Head of midle
10. Distal phalanx
11. Sesamoid bones
12. Trapezoid (Td)
13. Tubercle of trapezium
14. Capitate
15. Tubercle of scaphoid
16. Capitate (C)

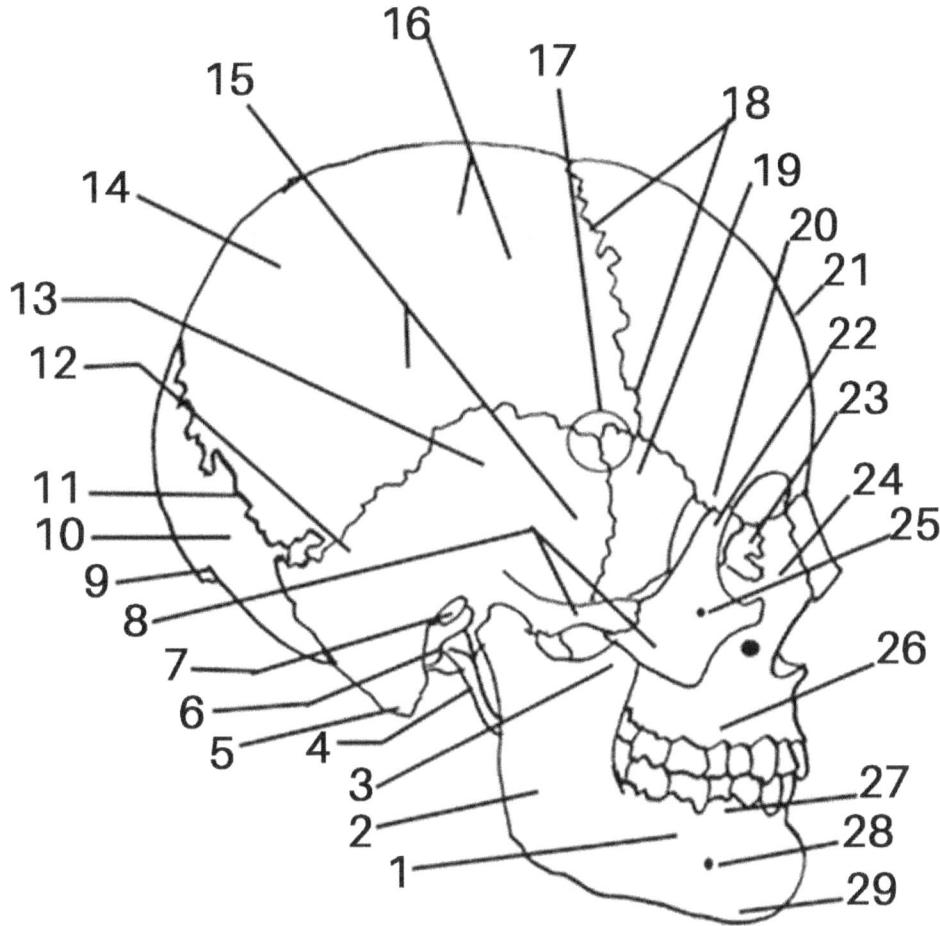

Adult cranium (Right Lateral Aspect)

1. Body of mandible
2. Rambus of mandible
3. Coronoid process of mandible
4. Styloid process of temporal bone
5. Mastoid process of temporal bone
6. Tympanic part of temporal bone
7. External acoustic meatus opening
8. Zygomatic process of temporal bobe
   Temporal process of zygomatic bone
9. External occipital protuberance (inion)
10. Superior nuchal line
11. Lambdoid suture
12. Mastoid part of temporal bone
13. Squaremous part of temporal bone
14. Region of parietal eminence
15. Temporal fossa
16. Superior & inferior Temporal lines
17. Pterion
18. Coronal suture
19. Temporal surface of greate wing of sphenoid
20. Zygomatic process of frontal bone
21. Frontal eminence
22. Frontal process of Zygomatic bone
23. Crest of lacrimal bone
24. Frontal process
25. Zygomaticofacial foramen
26. Alveolar process of maxilla
27. Alveolar part of mandible
28. Mental foramen
29. Mental tubercle

Bones of knee joint (Anterior View)

1. Fibula
2. Neck
3. Head
4. Apex of head
5. Lateral femorotibial articulation
6. Lateral femoral condyle
7. Lateral epicondyle
8. Patella
9. Femur
10. Q-angle
11. Head of femur
12. Anterior superior iliac spine (ASIS)
13. Femororpatellar
14. Adductor tubercle
15. Medial epicondyle
16. Medial Femoral condyle
17. Medial femorotibial articulation
18. Medial and lateral tibial condyles
19. Tuberosity
20. Axis of tibia
21. Tibia

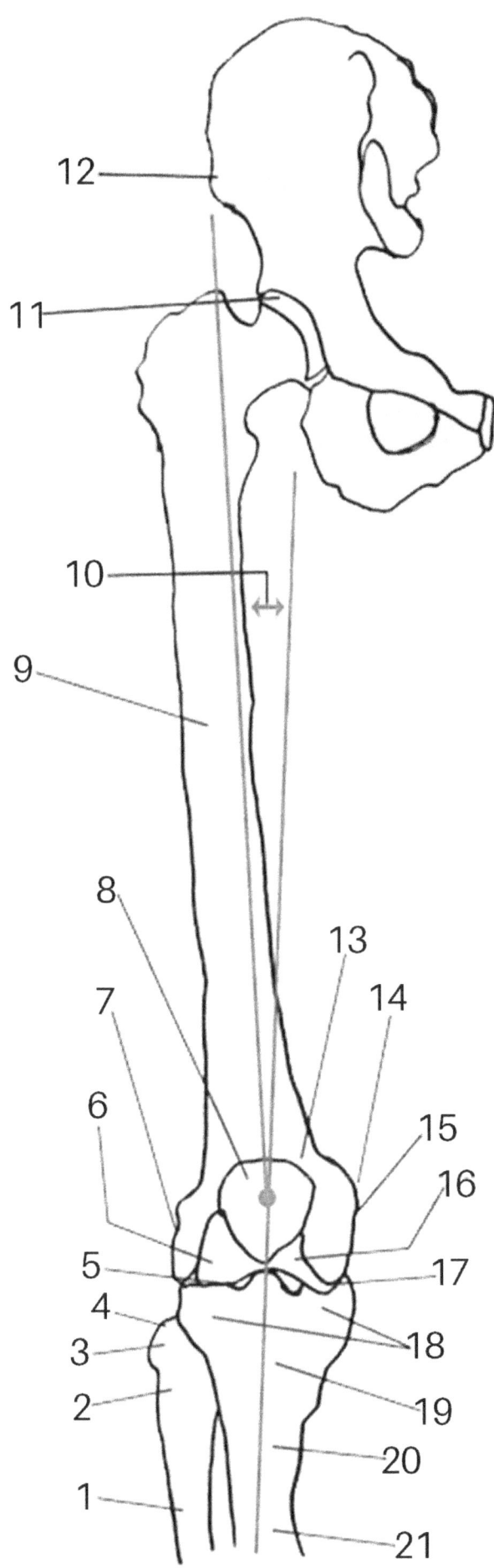

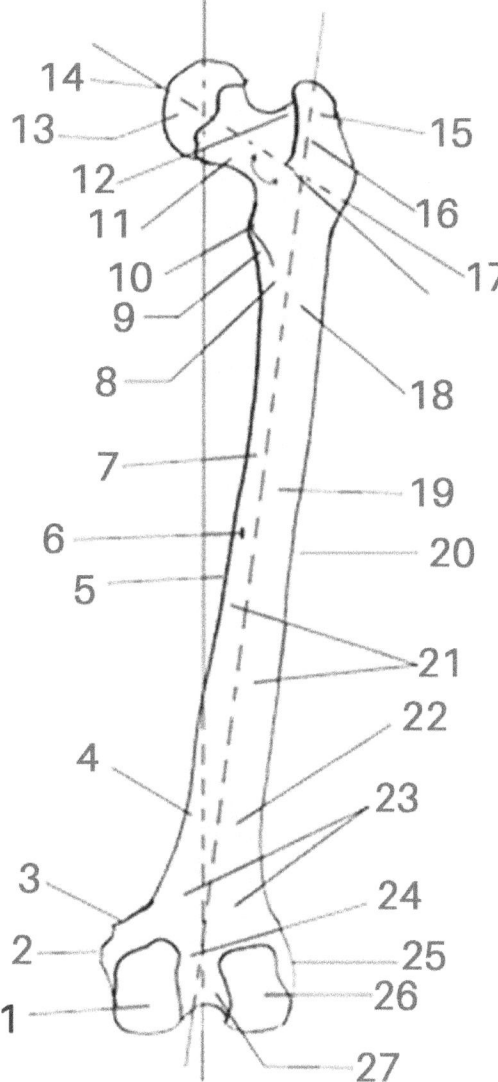

Right femur - Anterior View

1. Medial condyle
2. Medial epicondyle
3. Adductor tubercle
4. Medial supracondylar line
5. Nedial surface of shaft
6. Nutrient foramen
7. Medial lip of linea aspera
8. Spiral line
9. Pectineal line
10. Lesser trochanter
11. Neck
12. Trochanteric fossa
13. Head
14. Fovea for ligament of head
15. Greater trochanter
16. Quadrate tubercle
17. Intertrochanteric crest
18. Gluteal tuberosity
19. Lateral lip of linea aspera
20. Lateral surface of shaft
21. Posterior surface of shaft
22. Lateral supracondylar line
23. Popliteal surface
24. Intercondylar line
25. Lateral epicondyle
26. Lateral condyle
27. Intercondylar fossa

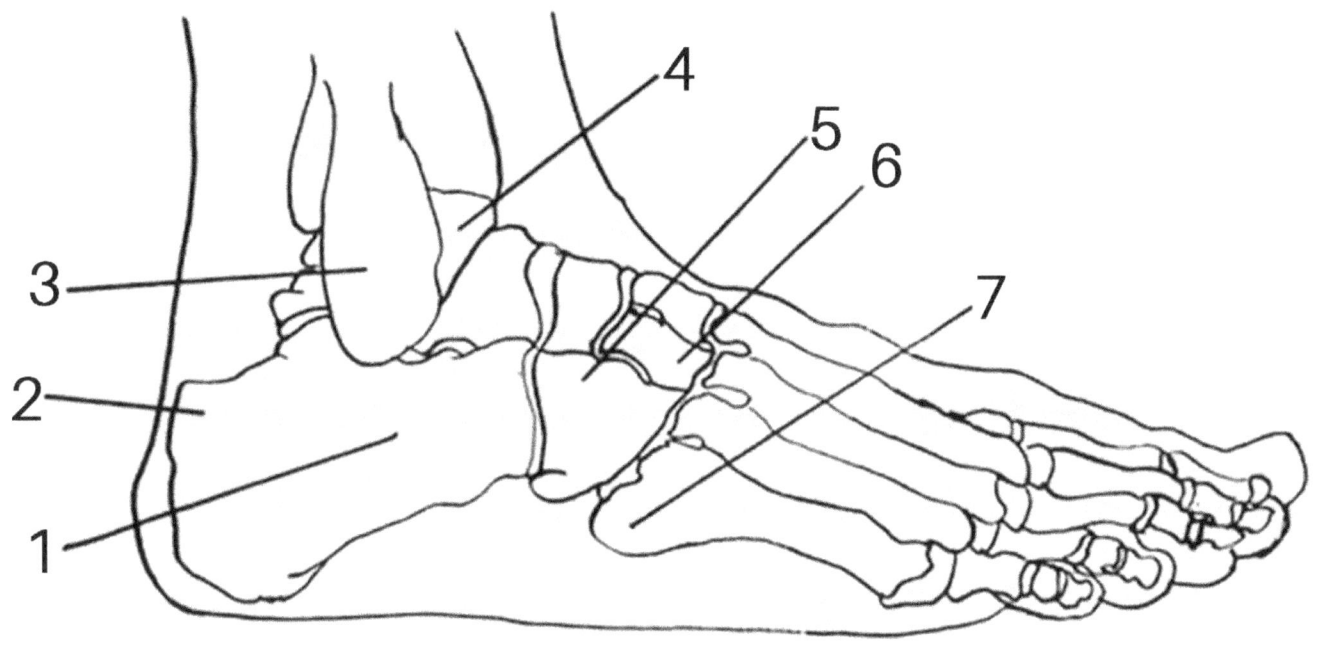

Surface projection and palpation of bony prominences of foot (Lateral Foot)

1. Fibular trochlea
2. Calcaneus
3. Lateral malleolus
4. Trochlea of talus
5. Cuboid
6. Lateral cuneiform
7. Tuberosity of 5th metatarsal

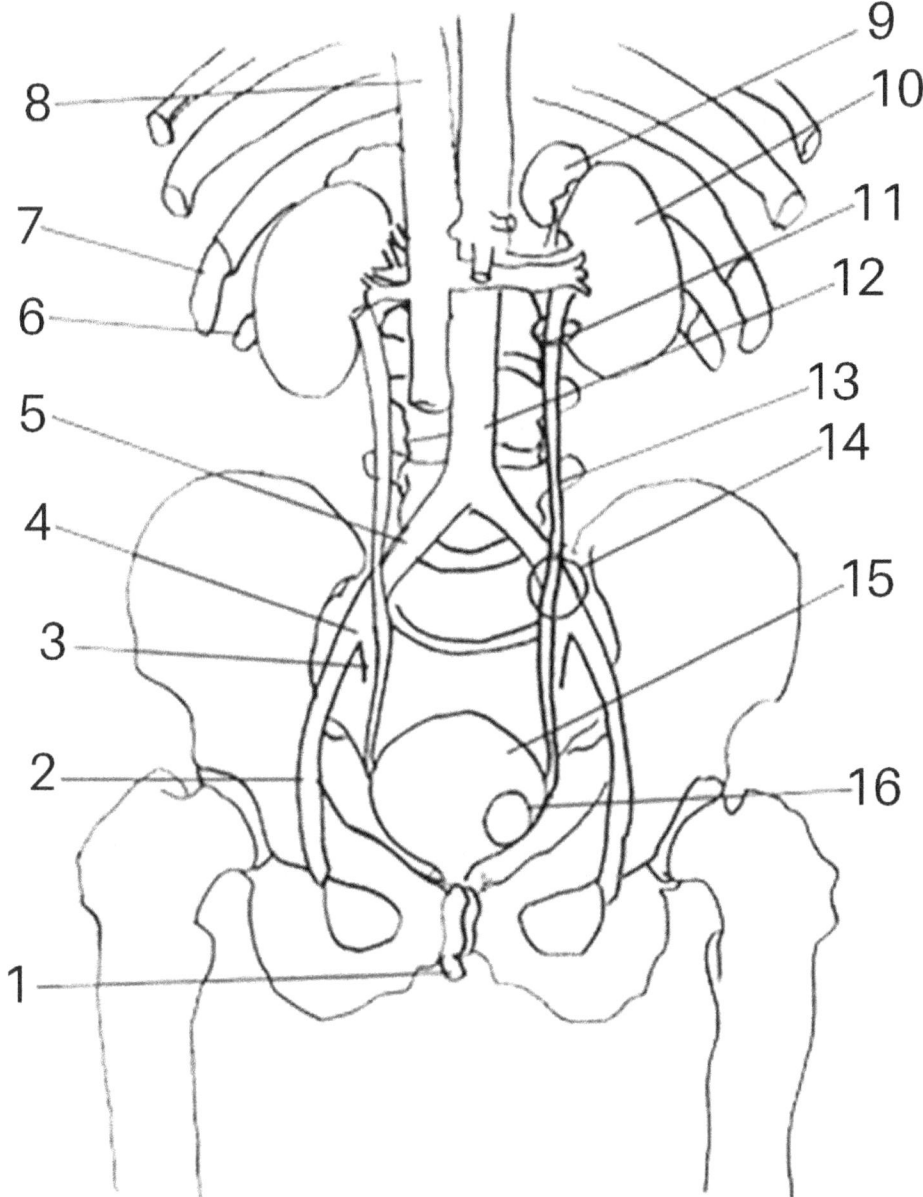

Genito-urinary viscera - Anterior View

1. Urethra
2. External iliac artery
3. Internal iliac artery
4. Bifurcation of common iliac artery
5. Common iliac artery
6. 12th rib
7. 11th rib
8. Inferior veba cava
9. Left suprarenal gland
10. Left kidney
11. Ureteropelvic junction
12. Abdominal aorta
13. Ureter
14. Crossing iliac vessels and pelvic brim
15. Urinary bladder
16. Trversing bladder wall

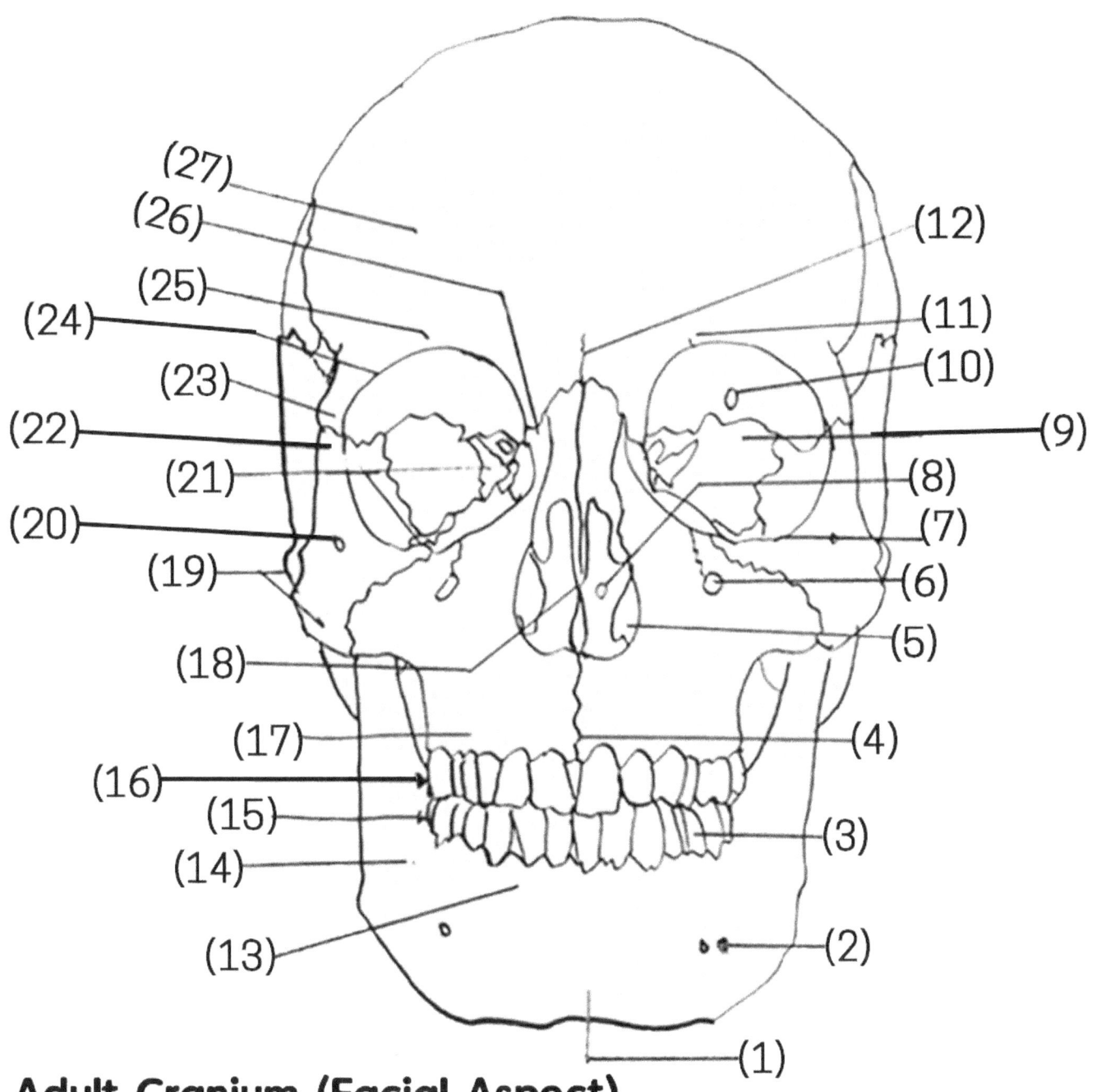

Adult Cranium (Facial Aspect)

1. Mental Protuberance
2. Mental Foramen
3. Premolar Teeth
4. Intermaxillary Suture
5. Inferior Nasal Concha
6. Infra-Orbital Foramen
7. Infra-Orbital Margin
8. Nasal Cavity
9. Orbital Surface of Greater wing of Sphenoid
10. Orbital Cavity
11. Supra-orbital foremen (notch)
12. Frontal (metopic) suture
13. Alveolar part of mandible
14. Oblique line
15. Mandibular teeth
16. Maxillary teeth
17. Alveolar process of maxilla
18. Nasal septum (bony part)
19. Zygomatic arc
20. Zygomaticofacial foramen
21. Superior & inferior orbital fissures
22. Frontal process of Zygomatic bone
23. Zygomatic Process
24. Supra-Orbital margin
25. Superciliary arch
26. Frontal process of Maxilla
27. Frontal Eminence

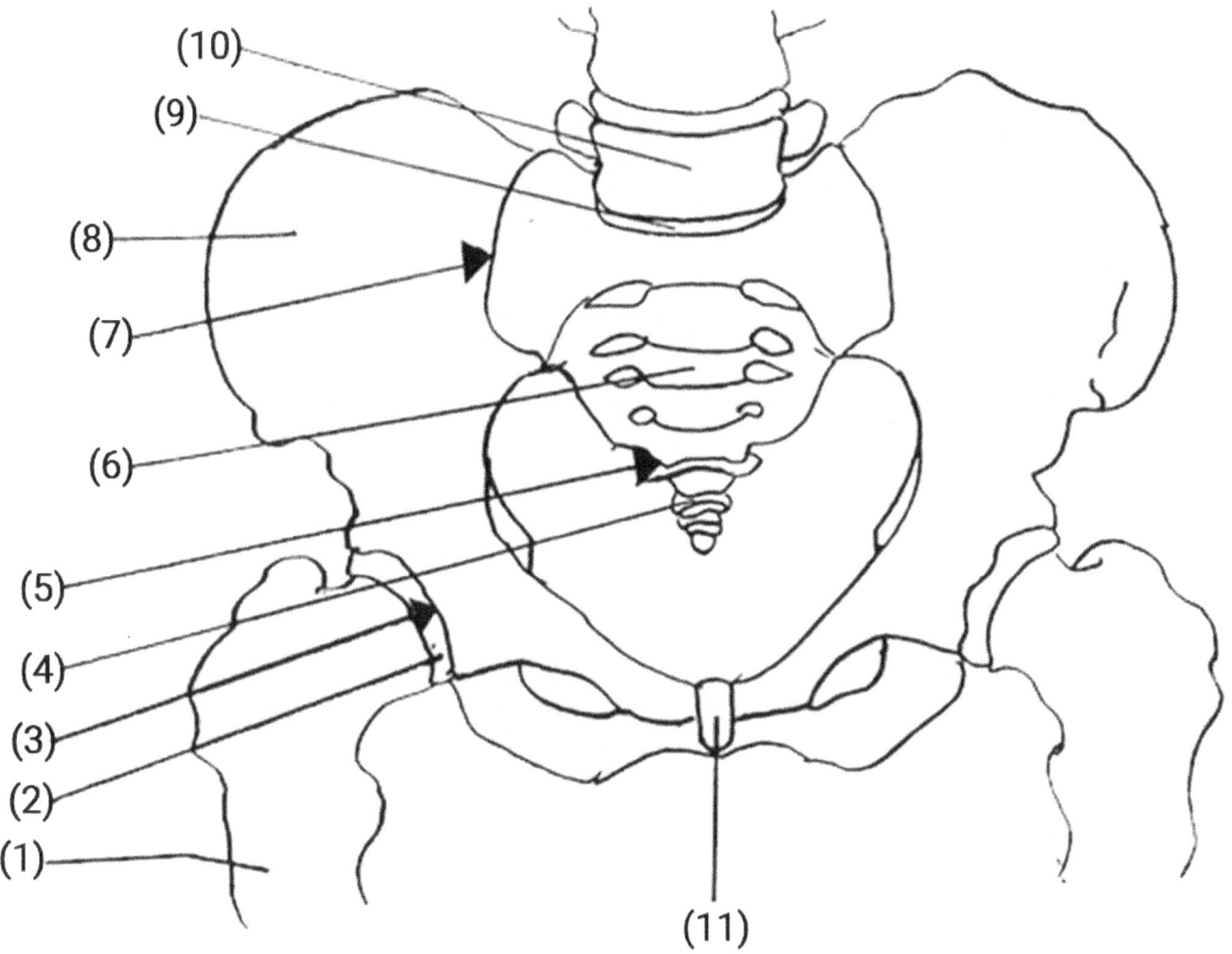

JOINTS OF PELVICE GIRDLE (ANTERIOR VIEW)

1. Femur
2. Head of Femur
3. Acetabulum
4. Coccyx
5. Sacro-Coccygeal Joint
6. Sacrum
7. Sacro-iliac joint
8. Ilium
9. Lumbosacral Joint
10. 5th lumbar vertebra (L5)
11. Pubic Symphysis

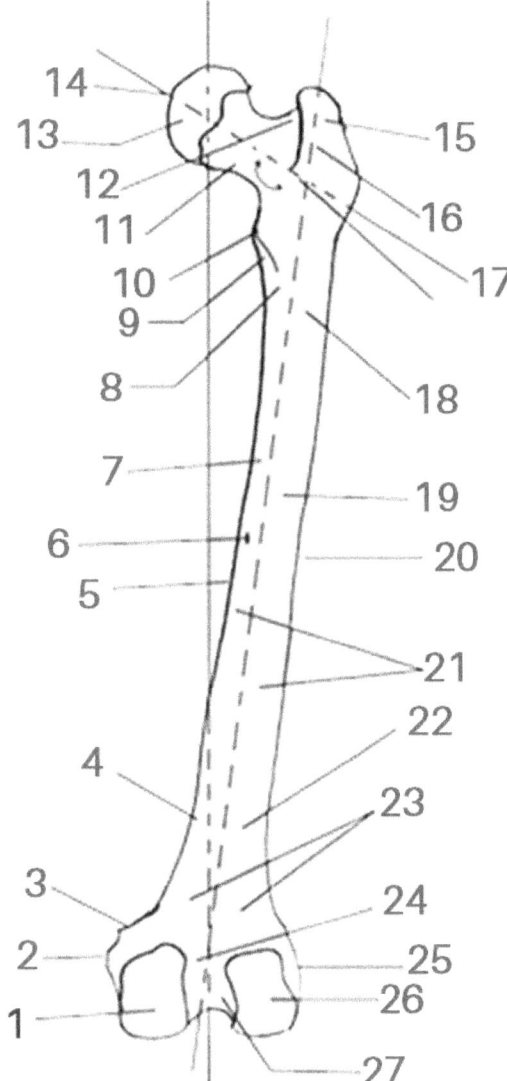

Right femur - Anterior View

1. Medial condyle
2. Medial epicondyle
3. Adductor tubercle
4. Medial supracondylar line
5. Medial surface of shaft
6. Nutrient foramen
7. Medial lip of linea aspera
8. Spiral line
9. Pectineal line
10. Lesser trochanter
11. Neck
12. Trochanteric fossa
13. Head
14. Fovea for ligament of head
15. Greater trochanter
16. Quadrate tubercle
17. Intertrochanteric crest
18. Gluteal tuberosity
19. Lateral lip of linea aspera
20. Lateral surface of shaft
21. Posterior surface of shaft
22. Lateral supracondylar line
23. Popliteal surface
24. Intercondylar line
25. Lateral epicondyle
26. Lateral condyle
27. Intercondylar fossa

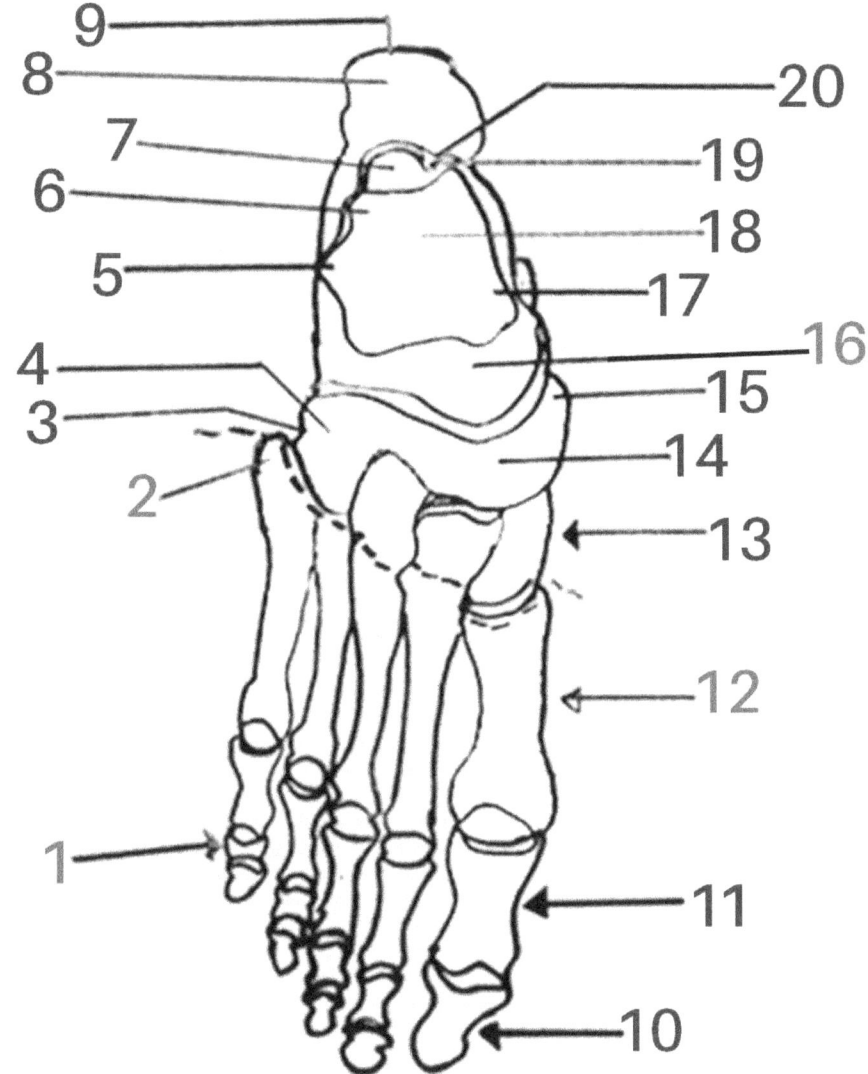

Bone of Right Foot

Superior View of Dorsum of foot

1. Middle phalanges
2. Tuberosity
3. Groove for fibularis longus
4. Cuboid
5. For lateral malleolus
6. Facet for inferior posterior tibiofibular ligament
7. Lateral tubercle
8. Calcaneus
9. Calcaneal tuberosity (posterior surface)
10. Distal phalanges
11. Proximal phalanges
12. Metatarsals
13. Cuneiforms
14. Navicular
15. Tuberosity
16. Talus
17. For medial malleolus
18. For tibia
19. Medial tubercle
20. Groove for flexor hallucis longus

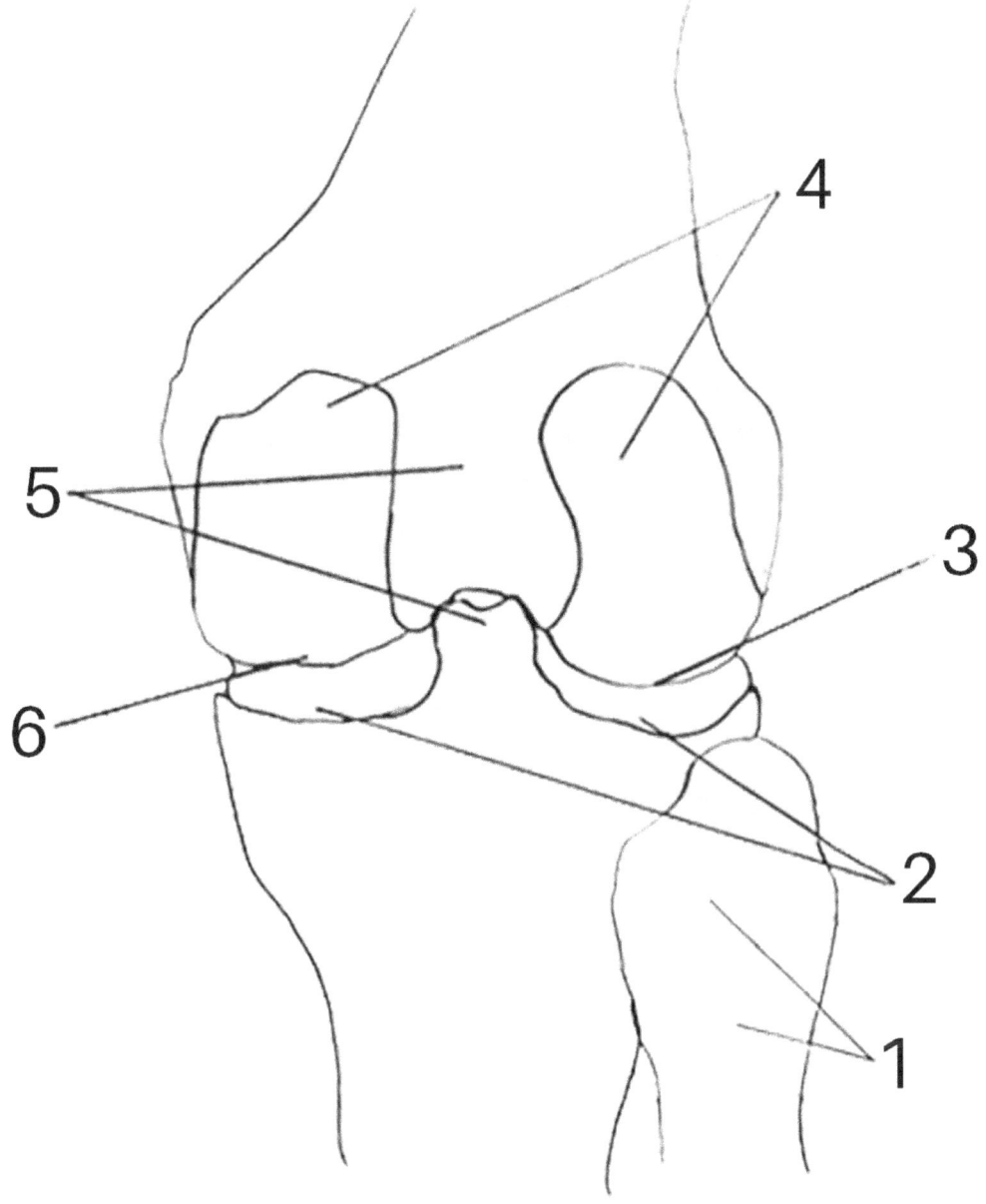

Bone of the Knee Joint (Posterior View)

1. Head and neck of fibula
2. Tibial condyles
3. Lateral femorotibial articulation
4. Femoral condyles
5. Intercondylar areas of femur and tibia
6. Medial femorotibial articulation

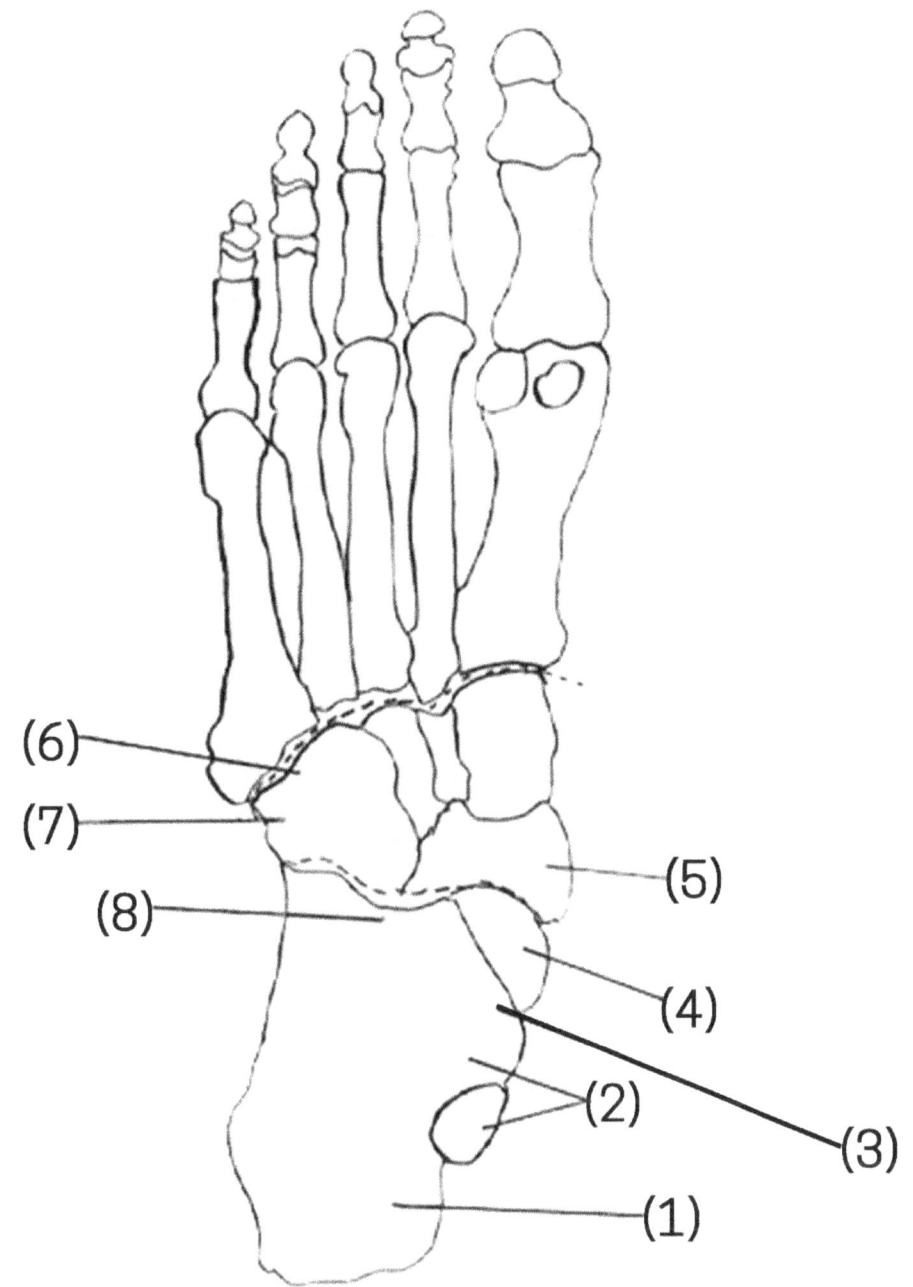

BONE OF RIGHT FOOT
(Inferior View of Plantar Aspect)

1. Calcaneus
2. Groove for flexor hallucis longus
3. Sustentaculum tali
4. Head of Talus
5. Navicular tuberosity
6. Groove for fibularis longus
7. Tuberosity of cuboid
8. Anterior tubercle

www.ingramcontent.com/pod-product-compliance
Lightning Source LLC
Chambersburg PA
CBHW080439220526
45465CB00009B/3354